The Healing Power of Power of Shea Butter

Unlocking Nature's Secret for Health and Wellness

By Charles Hardeyhorbah

TABLE OF CONTENTS

Introduction

The Rich Legacy of Shea Butter

The African shea tree (Vitellaria paradoxa) yields shea butter. The fat obtained from the shea nut is known as shea butter. Shea nuts are a naturally occurring, wild food that have been gathered and cooked for millennia in West and East African nations.

Shea butter naturally includes good-for-you ingredients like; Catechins, an antioxidant, and tocopherol, often known as vitamin E.Vitamins A and F, which have moisturizing and anti-aging effects

Shea butter contains a variety of fatty acids, including oleic, stearic, linoleic, and palmitic acids. These are great for the skin's barrier and enable the butter to mix in easily with your skin's natural oils.

This book explores the extraordinary qualities and countless advantages of shea butter. This book is a thorough reference that examines the long history of shea butter, its origins, and the research that underpins its therapeutic benefits.

For millennia, African tribes have used shea butter, which is made from the nuts of the shea tree, for both beauty and therapeutic uses. Shea butter has a wide range of health advantages that include skin care, hair care, wound healing, pain reduction, and more thanks to its special blend of vitamins, antioxidants, and vital fatty acids.

This book sets out on a historical journey to learn the origins of shea butter and its crucial function in African traditional medicine.It examines the cultural significance of shea butter, how it is made, and the groups of people who have protected this natural marvel for ages.

Taking a deeper look, this book explores the composition of shea butter, its abundance of vitamins A, E, and F, and its powerful antioxidants in order to reveal the intricate scientific details underlying the therapeutic powers of shea butter. You will learn in-depth information about how shea butter repairs, nourishes, and shields the body from outside threats through this investigation.

Sheabutter has particular uses for caring for skin, hair, and general wellbeing. In addition to its usefulness in reducing the symptoms of eczema and psoriasis, it can moisturize and revitalize the skin.It demonstrates that it is an adaptable and priceless ally in preserving good skin.

The book also discussed how shea butter can improve hair health by encouraging strength, gloss, and vitality.It reveals the mechanisms behind shea butter's success in promoting wound healing, minimizing scarring, and providing pain relief, demonstrating its promise as a natural substitute for conventional therapies.

It is impossible to overstate the value of shea butter for relaxation, aromatherapy, and lip care. It is crucial to a comprehensive approach to well-being because of its capacity to nourish, defend, and heal.

Along with a wealth of knowledge, "The Healing Power of Shea Butter" offers helpful advice, do-it-yourself recipes, and product suggestions. You will have a profound understanding of the healing powers of shea butter by the end of this book and the self-assurance to use it on a daily basis.

Chapter 1

The Origins of Shea Butter: A Natural Wonder

The women of the community gathered around the shea tree as the sun rose over the vast savannah, spreading a warm golden glow. They collected the ripe nuts, which contained the shea butter that was the key to their health and wellbeing, with deft hands. For centuries, they had relied on this marvel of nature, which was made from the nuts of the shea tree.

The shea tree, also known as Vitellaria paradoxa, is indigenous to the continent of Africa and is mainly found in the sub-Saharan areas. It comes from the nuts of karité trees that grow in the Sahel region extending from West to East Africa, from Guinea and Senegal to Uganda and South Sudan.

It is revered as the "tree of life," and with its roots firmly planted in African soil, it can survive in parched environments. The tree may reach a height of 15 meters and takes 20 years to produce its first crop.

The women of the community get together to gather the shea tree's fruits after it has blessed the land with them. The priceless kernel within is revealed after they delicately crack open the nuts. Shea butter is made from this fat-rich kernel. After roasting the kernels to give them a distinctive nutty flavor, the women ground and blend them into a smooth paste. They carefully follow a method to obtain the golden butter, which is then ready to be used for its numerous advantages.

During his travels in Africa in the 1790s, Scottish explorer Mungo Park wrote, "The natives were everywhere busy in collecting the fruit of the shea trees, from which they produce the vegetable butter

Shea butter has been a staple of African culture for many years. It is revered in conventional medicine because it is thought to have mystical characteristics. Shea butter is a gift that moms give to their daughters as a representation of the sage and nurturing nature of women.

Shea butter is mostly used in skincare products. Its high vitamin content, which includes vitamins A, E, and F, nourishes and hydrates the skin. Shea butter's emollient properties aid to lock in moisture, avoiding dryness and fostering a supple complexion. Because of its anti-inflammatory qualities, it is a useful treatment for calming sensitive skin disorders like eczema and dermatitis.

Shea butter also serves as a natural sunscreen, shielding skin from the damaging UV rays of the sun. Shea butter contains cinnamic acid, which offers a modest sun protection factor (SPF), protecting the skin from sunburn and early aging.

Shea butter has numerous health benefits for both the skin and hair. Its nourishing qualities penetrate the hair shaft deeply, hydrating and fortifying from the inside. Shea butter is a go-to product for those who want long, luscious hair since it reduces frizz, adds shine, and stimulates hair development.

Shea butter has been used for ages to treat wounds and ease joint and muscle discomfort in addition to its cosmetic uses. By lowering inflammation and avoiding infections, its anti-inflammatory and antibacterial characteristics support the healing process. Shea butter's high concentration of fatty acids, which includes oleic, stearic, and linoleic acids, encourages the creation of collagen and tissue regeneration, which reduces scarring.

Chapter 2

The Science Behind Shea Butter's Healing Properties

We learn the interesting science behind shea butter's incredible healing powers as we explore deeper into the product. Shea butter has long been regarded as a powerful natural treatment, but recent research has shed light on the exact ingredients and mechanisms that give it its reputation.

Several healthy substances, such as fatty acids, vitamins, and antioxidants are abundant in shea butter. Let's examine the scientific basis for each of these ingredients and how they contribute to the therapeutic effects of shea butter.

Vitamins are essential for preserving our skin's health and vibrancy. Vitamins A, E, and F are particularly rich in shea butter. Retinol, a form of vitamin A, encourages cell turnover and helps to enhance and revitalize skin.

Strong antioxidant vitamin E shields the skin from free radical-induced oxidative damage.

These toxic compounds are neutralized, preventing them from destroying the collagen and elastin fibers that are necessary for preserving the skin's suppleness and firmness. In addition to promoting a more even skin tone, vitamin E aids in the fading of scars and hyperpigmentation.

The vital fatty acid-containing vitamin F, which is less well-known, is crucial for maintaining the skin's barrier function. These fatty acids nourish and moisturize the skin, avoiding dryness and flakiness, and include linoleic acid and alpha-linolenic acid. Additionally, they have anti-inflammatory qualities that calm sensitive skin and lessen redness.

Another essential ingredient in shea butter that contributes to its therapeutic qualities is antioxidants. These potent substances aid in defending the skin from oxidative stress brought on by noxious substances, UV radiation, and pollution. Catechins, flavonoids, and triterpenes, among other antioxidants found in shea butter, collaborate to combat free radicals and promote skin health.

Cinnamic acid is one of the major antioxidants present in shea butter. Shea butter has a natural sun protection factor (SPF) of about 6 thanks to its ingredient. Shea butter provides an additional layer of defense against the sun's damaging UV rays, lowering the risk of sunburn and early aging even though it cannot replace a dedicated sunscreen product.

Shea butter is made up of fatty acids, which are essential to its medicinal qualities. Oleic acid, stearic acid, and linoleic acid are the three fatty acids that are most prevalent in shea butter. Shea butter can penetrate the skin and supply its nourishing properties thanks to oleic acid's deep moisturizing properties. Emollient qualities of stearic acid leave the skin feeling silky and soft. Linoleic acid can be especially helpful for people with acne-prone skin since it helps to maintain the skin's barrier function.

Shea butter's special blend of vitamins, antioxidants, and fatty acids works synergistically to offer a variety of advantages in addition to these individual components. It works well as a treatment for dry skin, eczema, psoriasis, and other inflammatory skin disorders because of its hydrating and anti-inflammatory characteristics. Shea butter's capacity to encourage collagen synthesis and tissue regeneration helps in scar healing, wound healing, and skin rejuvenation in general.

Our appreciation for shea butter's amazing therapeutic capabilities is increasing as our knowledge of its components and mechanisms deepens.

Chapter 3

Shea Butter and Skincare: Nourishing Your Body

In this chapter, we focus on one of shea butter's most popular and well-liked applications: skincare. Shea butter is a well-liked component in many skincare products due to its nourishing and moisturizing qualities, and a variety of skin problems can benefit from its natural goodness.

Shea Butter has a long history as a great skin care ingredient that reaches back to ancient Egypt. Pure, unrefined shea butter was something that Queen Cleopatra always had on hand.

One of shea butter's best qualities is its capacity to intensely hydrate and moisturize the skin. Shea butter is a fantastic option for battling dryness and preserving the best possible skin health since it contains a potent combination of fatty acids, vitamins, and antioxidants that assist to replace and retain moisture.

Dry skin can be irritating, flaking, and painful. Shea butter can be applied frequently to help skin regain moisture and form a barrier that keeps moisture in. Because of its abundant emollient qualities, the skin appears healthy and radiant and feels smooth, soft, and supple.

Shea butter helps to soothe and calm inflamed skin in addition to offering great hydration. Shea butter has anti-inflammatory ingredients including triterpenes and cinnamic acid that help lessen the redness, itching, and inflammation brought on by a variety of skin disorders. Shea butter can offer much-needed comfort and relief whether you have eczema, dermatitis, or just sensitive skin in general.

Shea butter contains vitamins that are essential for maintaining healthy skin. Retinol, a type of vitamin A, stimulates cell division and increases collagen synthesis. This can result in softer skin, less fine wrinkles, and an overall better complexion. Strong antioxidant vitamin E shields the skin from free radicals, aids in the lightening of scars and dark spots, and encourages a more uniform skin tone.

Sensitive skin sufferers might choose shea butter as well. For people who are prone to allergic reactions or skin irritations, it is a mild and safe solution due to its natural makeup and lack of harsh chemicals. It offers a nourishing and soothing moisturizer that can be used alone or as an ingredient in a variety of skincare products.

Shea butter's applicability goes beyond skincare for the face. It can be applied to the entire body, from head to toe, to hydrate and rejuvenate it. Shea butter can help replenish moisture, soften rough spots, and increase overall skin suppleness whether you have dry elbows and knees or rough heels.

Shea butter has advantages that are not just for adults; it is also gentle enough for baby and toddler skin. Its calming and nourishing qualities make it the perfect ingredient for baby care products since they assist to prevent diaper rash, calm inflamed skin, and prevent dryness..

It's crucial to select premium, unrefined shea butter when putting it into your skincare regimen. You will receive the greatest benefits if you use unrefined shea butter because it keeps its original color, scent, and beneficial qualities. Select shea butter from reliable vendors who promote fair trade and environmentally friendly business practices.

Chapter 4

Shea Butter for Hair Care: Strengthening and Repairing

The transforming potential of shea butter for hair care is explored in this chapter. Shea butter has earned its place as a favored ingredient in the pursuit of healthy and attractive hair thanks to its capacity to nourish and moisturize as well as its efficacy in controlling frizz and boosting hair growth.

Shea butter is a natural powerhouse for healthy hair thanks to its high content of fatty acids, vitamins, and antioxidants. By deeply hydrating dry and damaged hair, its moisturizing effects into the hair shaft. Shea butter may replenish moisture, making your hair softer, smoother, and easier to maintain whether your hair is naturally dry, has had chemical treatment, or has been exposed to environmental stressors.

Fighting frizzy hair can be a never-ending struggle, especially in humid weather. Shea butter saves the day by forming a layer of defense around the hair shaft, locking in moisture and halting the destructive effects of excessive humidity. The end effect is hair that is smoother, more under control, and less prone to frizz and flyaways.

Shea butter is an organic ally for encouraging hair development. Due to its nourishing qualities, hair follicles are strengthened, which lowers breakage and promotes healthy hair development. Shea butter contains vital vitamins and fatty acids that support the general health of the scalp and foster a favorable environment for hair growth.

The anti-inflammatory qualities of shea butter can also help people with scalp issues like dandruff or itching. Its calming and hydrating properties offer a healthy scalp and a stable environment for hair growth by easing itching and reducing inflammation.

There are various ways to integrate shea butter into your hair care routine. Shea butter is frequently used as a deep conditioner or hair mask. Simply warm up some shea butter in your hands and distribute it evenly through damp hair, paying special attention to the ends and any areas that require more hydration. For a highly nourishing treatment, leave it on for 20 to 30 minutes or even overnight. Then, carefully rinse.

Using shea butter-containing hair products is another approach to take use of its advantages. Look for shea butter in the formulations of shampoos, conditioners, leave-in treatments, and styling products. Your hair may receive constant hydration, protection, and manageability from these products.

Shea butter is especially helpful for people with curly or coily hair. Its thick texture aids in defining curls, taming frizz, and enhancing the natural texture. Apply creams, butters, or balms with shea butter as the primary ingredient to damp or dry hair to create desired styles while keeping curls hydrated and bouncy.

The important fatty acids linoleic acid and oleic acid, both of which help moisturize and nourish the hair and are crucial in preventing hair loss, are abundant in shea butter. Additionally, these fatty acids aid in enhancing blood flow to the scalp, which encourages the development of thick, healthy hair.

Shea butter should be applied sparingly because excessive amounts can weigh down delicate hair or leave an oily residue. Start with a tiny quantity and titrate as necessary for your hair.

Chapter 5

Shea Butter for Wound Healing: Nature's Remedy

Shea butter is remarkably effective at speeding up the healing of wounds. Shea butter has been valued for its therapeutic qualities throughout history, and contemporary research is still revealing more of this potential. Shea butter can be an all-natural and efficient ally in the healing process for anything from minor cuts and abrasions to more serious wounds.

Shea butter's special blend of fatty acids, vitamins, and antioxidants aids in its capacity to heal wounds. The fatty acids nourish and hydrate the afflicted area, while the presence of vitamins A and E aids skin regeneration and restoration. The anti-inflammatory properties of shea butter also aid in reducing inflammation and fostering a favorable environment for healing.

Shea butter creates a barrier of protection around the wounded region when it is applied to wounds. This barrier prevents external irritants, bacteria, and pollutants from entering the wound, lowering the risk of infection and accelerating the healing process. Shea butter's hydrating qualities also keep the wound from drying out, which can cause scabbing and a slower rate of healing.

Shea butter contains triterpenes, which further promotes wound healing. Triterpenes have anti-inflammatory and antibacterial qualities that aid to relax surrounding tissue and guard against potential infection. Shea butter minimizes swelling and discomfort by lowering inflammation, which improves the effectiveness of the body's built-in healing processes.

Shea butter's soothing and moisturizing qualities are essential in reducing scarring. Shea butter aids in promoting the growth of healthy tissue and reducing the formation of scar tissue by keeping the wound hydrated and preventing excessive dryness. This may lead to less obvious scarring and a more attractive outcome.

Start by washing the injured area completely with mild soap and water before applying shea butter for wound healing. Apply a thin layer of shea butter directly to the wound or the surrounding skin after gently patting the area dry. Make sure your hands are clean to avoid spreading any more bacteria. Repeat this procedure as necessary, at least twice daily, while keeping an eye on the healing of the wound.

While shea butter might be helpful for minor wounds and abrasions, it's crucial to keep in mind that more serious injuries might necessitate medical treatment. To receive an accurate diagnosis and advice for treatment, speak with a healthcare expert.

Shea butter speeds up the healing process for cuts, abrasions, and other wounds because it contains vitamins and phytonutrients that are absorbed into the skin's subcutaneous tissue. Nothing absorbs as deeply into the skin as Shea butter, which helps wounds heal from the inside out.

Shea butter not only heals wounds but also soothes and relieves various skin irritations like burns, bug bites, and rashes. Its anti-inflammatory and moisturizing qualities offer relief and speed up healing.

Shea butter's versatility as a natural remedy never ceases to astound, and one of its many amazing uses is in the treatment of wounds.

Chapter 6

Shea Butter for Dry and Sensitive Skin: Restoring Balance and Comfort

This chapter explores shea butter's healing and calming effects on dry, sensitive skin. Shea butter can offer the much-needed relief and restoration your skin yearns for, whether you deal with persistently dry skin or occasionally feel irritation.

Itchy, unpleasant, and prone to flaking, dry skin can be. Shea butter works as a natural moisturizer, nourishing the skin from the inside out and assisting in its return to its smoothness and suppleness. Because of the high concentration of fatty acids in it, particularly oleic, stearic, and linoleic acids, the skin's surface is protected, keeping moisture in and avoiding moisture loss. The skin's natural lipid barrier, which is crucial for preserving proper moisture, is restored with the aid of this barrier.

Shea butter has the capacity to provide long-lasting hydration, which is one of the reasons it is very advantageous for dry skin.

Shea butter's emollient properties penetrate the skin deeply, nourishing and hydrating from inside, in contrast to certain moisturizers that only offer momentary relief. Shea butter can help the skin retain moisture better over time, reducing dryness and producing a more youthful, hydrated appearance.

Skin that is sensitive needs special care and consideration. Shea butter is a great option for people with sensitive skin because of how soothing and non-irritating it is. It is suitable for even the most delicate skin types because it doesn't include any harsh chemicals or scents that can cause reactions. The natural properties of shea butter relax and soothe inflamed skin, reducing redness, irritation, and inflammation.

Like an emollient, shea butter works. It could aid in softer or smoother dry skin. Shea butter also has ingredients that might lessen skin edema. This could be used to treat skin-swelling disorders including eczema.

Shea butter has various ingredients that make it useful for dry and sensitive skin in addition to its hydrating qualities. Triterpenes, which have anti-inflammatory qualities, assist in reducing the redness and inflammation brought on by sensitive skin disorders like rosacea or eczema. Cinnamic acid, a phenolic molecule, has anti-aging and antioxidant properties that help the skin look younger by shielding it from free radical damage.

Choose products with shea butter as a primary component to include shea butter in your skincare regimen for dry and sensitive skin. Look for high-quality shea butter in gentle cleansers, moisturizers, and serums. These formulas can aid in skin renewal and hydration, relieving dryness and fostering a balanced, healthy complexion.

Pure shea butter can be applied directly to the problematic areas for focused treatment of particularly dry or sensitive areas, such as elbows, knees, or spots of eczema. Shea butter's nourishing properties will work their magic if you gently massage a small bit of it into your skin until it is completely absorbed.

It's crucial to remember that each person has a different type of skin, so what works for one person might not work for another. A dermatologist or skincare expert can provide you with tailored recommendations if you have particular issues or medical conditions.

Chapter 7

Shea Butter for Lip Care: Nourishing and Protecting Your Smile

The advantages of shea butter for lip care are discussed in this chapter. Because our lips are frequently exposed to severe environmental factors, they are prone to becoming dry, chapped, and unpleasant. Shea butter is a fantastic option for preserving soft, smooth, and healthy lips because of its moisturizing and nourishing qualities.

Sebaceous glands, which normally create oils to keep the skin hydrated, are absent from the delicate skin of our lips. Our lips are more vulnerable to dryness and dehydration as a result. With its capacity to offer strong hydration and moisture retention, shea butter comes to the rescue. The delicate skin of the lips is replenished and restored by its high content of fatty acids, vitamins, and antioxidants, avoiding dryness and maintaining optimal lip health.

The emollient qualities of shea butter produce a barrier of protection that keeps moisture on the lips and prevents moisture loss. This barrier lessens the likelihood of chapping and cracking by protecting the lips from abrasive weather elements including dry air and chilly breezes. Shea butter helps keep your lips smooth, supple, and kissable with regular application.

Shea butter contains vitamins, such as vitamins A and E, which help to maintain the general health and wellbeing of your lips. Vitamin E functions as a powerful antioxidant, shielding the lips from free radicals and environmental damage, while vitamin A serves to boost cell turnover and encourage the formation of new, healthy skin cells. These vitamins function as a team to maintain the healthiest possible lips.

People with sensitive or inflamed lips can also benefit from shea butter's inherent anti-inflammatory qualities. Shea butter can help relax and soothe the skin, whether your lips are irritated from excessive licking, sunburn, or cold sores. It is suitable for people with sensitive skin or those who have allergic reactions to specific lip care products due to its mild and non-irritating nature.

Look for lip balms or other lip care items that include shea butter as a primary ingredient to include it to your routine. Shea butter benefits will be included in these formulas along with other elements that are good for lips. Apply the lip balm before bedtime and during the day, especially in dry or cold conditions, to keep your lips moisturized and protected.

Making your own shea butter lip balm at home is an option if you prefer a do-it-yourself strategy. Melt some shea butter with other nutritious ingredients like beeswax, coconut oil, and a tiny bit of your preferred essential oil for scent. The substance should be heated before being poured into lip balm containers to set. You'll be prepared with a handmade lip balm to maintain the health and moisture of your lips.

To keep your body and lips moisturized from the inside out, don't forget to drink lots of water throughout the day. Avoid excessive lip-licking since saliva can exacerbate dryness and irritation of the skin. When outdoors, use lip balm with SPF or wear a hat with a wide brim

to shield your lips from the sun's harmful UV
rays.

Chapter 8

Shea Butter for Overall Well-Being: Nurturing Body and Mind

Shea butter has all-encompassing advantages for general wellbeing. Shea butter can benefit your self-care regimen, encourage relaxation, and nourish your body and mind in addition to its outward uses.

Shea butter has the ability to ease muscle pains and stress, which is one way it improves general health. Its calming and anti-inflammatory qualities might ease aching muscles brought on by physical effort, exercise, or daily activities. Shea butter is frequently used by massage therapists in their treatments to assist the body unwind and regenerate. Shea butter's silky texture makes it simple to use and glide over the skin, improving the massage sensation.

Shea butter cream aids in the treatment of muscle discomfort, which can cause the body to become inflamed and rigid. Due to its anti-inflammatory and analgesic qualities, it aids in reducing swelling and pain in muscles. Your skin will retain a clear layer that is perfect for relaxation and your well-being. Your skin will feel quite soft once it is all finished. Shea butter can be used as a massage oil to ease tension in your muscles, similar to hydrating lotions.

Shea butter not only has health advantages for the body but also for the mind. Its natural aroma, which is frequently characterized as earthy and nutty, helps relax the senses. You can induce a state of calm and mindfulness by performing a shea butter self-massage routine. Take deep breaths and allow yourself to be present in the moment as you slowly massage the shea butter into your skin, relishing a sensation of serenity and wellbeing.

You can use shea butter in a variety of ways as part of your self-care routine. Shea butter can be combined with other nutritious oils like coconut oil, jojoba oil, or sweet almond oil to make a delightful body butter. This self-made body butter

You can use shea butter in a variety of ways as part of your self-care routine. Shea butter can be combined with other nutritious oils like coconut oil, jojoba oil, or sweet almond oil to make a delightful body butter. After taking a bath or shower, you may use this homemade body butter to lock in moisture and leave your skin feeling silky smooth.

Consider utilizing shea butter as a primary component in a homemade foot lotion for a revitalizing and hydrating foot treatment. Massage shea butter over your feet, giving special attention to any dry or hard areas. Combine shea butter with essential oils recognized for their calming effects, such lavender or peppermint. This self-care routine can bring about both physical and mental relief. Shea butter has a variety of uses, including aromatherapy. Shea butter's natural aroma can be improved by combining it with essential oils that go well with its earthy undertones. For promoting relaxation and stress reduction, lavender, chamomile, or ylang-ylang essential oils are wonderful options. You can include the advantages of shea butter into your wellness routines by making your own aromatherapy products using shea butter, like a calming body lotion or a calming massage oil.

As with any form of self-care, it's crucial to pay attention to your body and discover what works best for you. Shea butter can be used in a variety of ways, so experiment to find out what soothes and relaxes you the best. Include shea butter in your regular self-care regimen and benefit from its nourishing properties.

Chapter 9

Shea Butter for Skin Health: Nurturing Radiance and Vitality

Shea butter has remarkable advantages for the health of the skin.Shea butter has exceptional qualities that go beyond moisturizing to support brightness, energy, and general skin health. Let's look at how this all-natural component can give you a complexion that is radiant and youthful.

Shea butter has a high vitamin content, including vitamins A and E, which helps to nourish and renew the skin. Vitamin A helps to increase cell renewal, stimulate collagen synthesis, and lessen the visibility of fine lines and wrinkles. Additionally, it helps the skin maintain its natural suppleness, making it appear firmer and younger. A potent antioxidant, vitamin E shields the skin from environmental stresses and free radicals that can speed up the aging process.

Shea butter's blend of fatty acids, including oleic and stearic acids, contributes to the replenishment and restoration of the skin's moisture barrier. Shea butter helps to maintain ideal levels of hydration by locking in moisture, reducing dryness, and producing a plump and supple skin. Shea butter use on a regular basis can help create a skin barrier that is more resilient and well-balanced, reducing irritation and enhancing overall skin health.

Because of its inherent emollient qualities, shea butter is a fantastic product for anyone with dry or rough skin. Because of its rich structure, it may penetrate the skin deeply and give long-lasting hydration and suppleness. Applying shea butter on a regular basis can help address skin issues like dry patches, rough elbows, and cracked heels. This promotes softer, more touchable skin.

Shea butter has some special properties, one of which is its capacity to simultaneously treat various skin issues. In people with oily or mixed skin, it can help balance oil production by lowering excess sebum while supplying necessary hydration. Shea butter is suitable for people who are prone to breakouts or acne because it is non-comedogenic, which means it is unlikely to clog pores. In addition, its anti-inflammatory characteristics can help calm and soothe sensitive skin, offering relief from disorders like rosacea or eczema.

Choose skincare products with high-quality shea butter as a main ingredient if you want to incorporate shea butter for overall skin health. Look for skin moisturizers, serums, or masks that combine shea butter's moisturizing properties with additional advantageous components. These products can aid with skin texture, encourage a healthy complexion, and provide your skin the vital nutrients it requires to thrive.

Pure shea butter can be applied as a spot treatment to target specific regions, such as dry patches or fine wrinkles. Shea butter can be applied to the desired location by gently warming a tiny quantity between your hands and kneading it in until absorbed. Wake up to skin that has been renewed and regenerated by letting the shea butter do its magic over the course of the night.

When incorporating shea butter into your skincare routine, keep in mind that consistency is essential. Shea butter advantages can be maximized and your skin's health and appearance can be long-term improved with regular usage of shea butter. Before using shea butter, as with any skincare product, it's crucial to conduct a patch test, especially if you have sensitive skin or a history of allergies.

Chapter 10

Shea Butter in Natural Beauty Formulations: Harnessing Nature's Goodness

Due of its remarkable qualities, shea butter is a preferred component in many skincare, haircare, and body care products. Let's explore how shea butter might improve the efficacy and advantages of all-natural cosmetic products.

Shea butter has several beneficial properties in natural beauty products, one of which is its capacity to deliver intense and long-lasting hydration. Shea butter aids in retaining moisture when added to creams, lotions, or body butters, preventing moisture loss and preserving the skin's normal moisture levels. As a result, it is a useful element for those with dry or dehydrated skin since it provides nourishing and suppleness over the long term.

Shea butter improves the texture and spreadability of natural beauty treatments in addition to its hydrating effects. Because of its simple application and sumptuous, velvety feel, it has a smooth, creamy consistency. Shea butter aids in forming a barrier of protection on the skin, ensuring that the formulation's active components are adequately distributed and absorbed.

Shea butter's abundant concentration of fatty acids, vitamins, and antioxidants improves natural beauty products in a variety of ways. These organic substances support the overall health and happiness of the skin and hair. Shea butter enhances the manageability and gloss of hair strands, moisturizes the scalp, and encourages the growth of healthy hair when used in haircare products.

Shea butter is a fantastic component in lip balms, lip scrubs, and lip masks due to its nourishing and protecting qualities. Shea butter can hydrate and soften the sensitive skin on the lips, preventing chapping, drying, and cracking. Your lips will feel exceptionally soft and kissable thanks to its natural emollient characteristics, which produce a smooth and supple texture.

Shea butter is suitable for facial skincare formulations because it is non-comedogenic, especially for people with sensitive or acne-prone skin. It lessens the likelihood of breakouts by maintaining the skin's moisture balance without clogging pores. Shea butter is advantageous for those with illnesses like rosacea or eczema because of its anti-inflammatory characteristics, which can help calm and soothe sensitive skin.

Finding high-quality, sustainably sourced shea butter is essential when choosing natural beauty products that use it. Choose shea butter-based products that are unrefined or raw since they retain the most healthy nutrients and useful components. Think about endorsing companies that value fair trade relationships with shea butter growers and ethical sourcing methods.

Shea butter can be a satisfying ingredient to use in homemade recipes for people who like a do-it-yourself approach to beauty. The options are infinite, ranging from body butters and facial masks to hair treatments and lip balms. Create individualized cosmetic formulations that are tailored to your unique needs by experimenting with various combinations of natural components, such as essential oils, botanical extracts, or carrier oils.

You may embrace the power of nature in your daily self-care rituals thanks to shea butter's adaptability in natural beauty products. Shea butter's extraordinary characteristics will leave your skin, hair, and body feeling nourished, energized, and radiantly attractive whether you decide to indulge in store-bought products or explore the world of DIY beauty.

Chapter 11

Shea Butter for Hair Health: Nurturing Luscious Locks

Shea butter has restorative qualities that go beyond skin care; they may also do wonders for your hair, enhancing its vigor, strength, and general health. Learn how shea butter can become your hair's closest friend in the following paragraphs.

Shea butter's extraordinary ability to moisturize hair is one of its main benefits. Hair that is dry and brittle can be caused by a number of things, including chemical treatments, heat styling, and environmental damage. Shea butter helps to replenish moisture to the hair shaft by containing a high concentration of fatty acids and vitamins, which prevents frizz, dryness, and breaking. Shea butter can make your hair feel profoundly nourished, silky, and manageable when used frequently.

Shea butter is a fantastic option for people with damaged or unruly hair because it also has natural emollient properties. Shea butter coats each hair strand thanks to its creamy texture, leaving a smooth, protective layer behind. This gives your hair a natural sheen, controls frizz, and locks in moisture. Bid farewell to flyaways and welcome to lush, well-groomed hair.

Shea butter not only moisturizes but also strengthens the hair shaft, lowering the chance of breakage and split ends. Shea butter contains vitamins A and E, which nourish the scalp and support the hair follicles to encourage the growth of healthy hair. Shea butter may do wonders for your hair, whether you're trying to achieve longer hair or just want to improve the condition of it overall.

Shea butter may be found in a variety of hair care products thanks to its adaptability. Look for shea butter as a main ingredient in shampoos, conditioners, and hair treatments. These formulas make use of the advantages of shea butter to effectively cleanse and condition the hair. Hair creams and leave-in conditioners with shea butter as an ingredient provide your hair extra nourishment and defense all day long.

Use shea butter as a hair mask for a deeply hydrating and rejuvenating treatment. Shea butter may be easily melted and used liberally to your hair, paying special attention to the ends and damaged regions. For a more thorough treatment, leave the mask on for at least 30 minutes or overnight. Rinse completely, then take pleasure in its velvety smoothness.

Curls can also be tamed and defined using shea butter. Its hydrating qualities work to tame frizz and bring out your curls' organic texture. Apply a tiny amount of shea butter to damp hair after washing and conditioning it, scrunching it upwards to promote the production of curls. For defined, bouncy curls, let your hair air dry or use a diffuser.

It's crucial to select shea butter products that are of the highest caliber and are unrefined when utilizing shea butter in your haircare regimen. This makes sure you are getting the most out of this amazing ingredient. Additionally, watch how much shea butter you use because too much might make your hair heavy. Start off small and increase or decrease as necessary.

You may nurture and make your hair into the crowning glory of beauty and health with shea butter as your ally. Enjoy the luscious locks

you've always wanted and embrace the natural
goodness of shea butter.

Chapter 12

Sustainable Shea Butter: Empowering Communities, Preserving Nature

This chapter delves further into the vital subject of ethical sourcing and production methods in the shea butter sector. We examine the significance of these methods for the protection of the environment as well as the empowerment and welfare of the people involved in the production of shea butter.

The shea tree, or Vitellaria paradoxa as it is named scientifically, is the main source of shea butter. These trees are indigenous to the West African savannah regions of Africa. Communities in these areas have relied on the extraction and processing of shea butter for decades, especially the women who are principally in charge of its production.

Sustainable sourcing methods call for the environmentally friendly production and harvesting of shea nuts. It includes techniques for preserving biodiversity, stopping deforestation, and safeguarding the shea tree population. Sustainable business practices guarantee the long-term availability of this priceless resource by protecting the shea trees' natural habitat.

The promotion of agroforestry practices is one element of sustainable shea butter production. Shea trees are planted along with other crops, including vegetables or cereals, in agroforestry. Shea trees develop sustainably under this integrated method because they profit from their interactions with other plants and contribute to the ecosystem's overall health, which helps farmers diversify their sources of income.

Sustainable sourcing places a strong emphasis on fair trade values and equitable business relationships in addition to agricultural methods. It focuses on giving local communities economic opportunity and making sure they are fairly compensated for their labor. Sustainable business practices can improve the lifestyles of shea butter producers by developing transparent supply chains and fair trade agreements, enabling them to live more wealthy and sustainable lives.

Environmentally responsible extraction and processing techniques are also used in the production of sustainable shea butter. Shea nuts are gathered, dried, and pounded to separate the butter in traditional methods of shea butter extraction. By adopting cutting-edge technology that boost efficiency while reducing their negative effects on the environment, sustainable practices seek to optimize these processes.

Shea butter extraction from the nuts using mechanical presses is one such breakthrough. The labor-intensive pounding procedure is reduced by mechanical pressing, which also provides higher yields with less energy use. Additionally, these contemporary techniques frequently include filtration techniques to get rid of contaminants and raise the caliber of the shea butter.

Quality assurance and adherence to international standards are given priority in sustainable sourcing and production methods. This entails making sure that shea butter is made under sanitary circumstances, free from impurities or adulterants. Sustainable shea butter achieves market acceptance by conforming to these requirements, opening doors for ethical and fair trade collaborations with cosmetic and beauty industries.

Look for certifications like Fairtrade, Organic, or Rainforest Alliance, which show commitment to sustainable practices and fair trade standards, when purchasing shea butter goods. You may help to protect the environment and the well-being of the communities engaged in the production of shea butter by patronizing businesses that place a high priority on sustainability.

Chapter 13

Shea Butter in Everyday Life: Practical Tips and Applications

The practical aspects of incorporating shea butter into your everyday life and beauty routine are covered in this chapter. Shea butter's adaptability enables it to be utilized in numerous products other than skincare and haircare. Let's look at some original and useful strategies for using shea butter in your daily life.

1. Shea butter is an excellent natural treatment for dry and chapped lips. Shea butter and beeswax may be melted together to make your own lip balm, which can then be scented with a few drops of your favorite essential oil. Use this homemade lip balm frequently to maintain your lips kissable, soft, and hydrated.

2. Healing and Nourishing Cuticles. Shea butter can be used to your cuticles to moisturize them and keep them from drying out or splitting. This easy technique might help give your hands and nails a healthier appearance.

3. Softening Dry, Rough regions Like Elbows and Heels: Shea butter's thick texture makes it a great emollient for dry, rough regions like elbows and heels. Before going to bed, apply shea butter to these spots and let it work its magic all night. The texture and tenderness of these rough places will noticeably soften with continued application.

4. Nurturing and Protecting Baby's Skin. To maintain your child's skin supple, smooth, and well-hydrated, use shea butter as a natural moisturizer. It's also a great choice for treating diaper rash or dry skin spots on babies.

5.Shea butter can be used as a carrier oil in massage and aromatherapy, which enhances both practices. While being applied, its moisturizing qualities nurture the skin because of its smooth texture. Shea butter can be combined with a few drops of your preferred essential oils for a calming and fragrant experience.

6. Taming Flyaways and Frizzy Hair: Shea butter can be used as a natural hair styling product to get rid of flyaways and frizz. To tame unruly strands and add luster, simply spread a

tiny bit of shea butter over your hair while rubbing it between your palms. Curly or textured hair responds extremely well to this treatment.

7. Make-Your-Own Body Butter: Blend shea butter with additional nutritious ingredients to make your own opulent body butter. Melt shea butter and combine it with your chosen carrier oil, such as coconut, jojoba, or olive oil. For aroma, stir in a few drops of essential oils and allow the mixture to harden. Use this homemade body butter to treat yourself and really hydrate your body.

8. After-Sun Care: Shea butter is a great option for after-sun care because to its calming and hydrating qualities. Shea butter can help restore moisture and calm any burnt or irritated skin by being applied to sun-exposed regions. Its built-in anti-inflammatory abilities help relieve pain and speed up recovery.

To keep your shea butter consistent and of high quality, store it somewhere cold and dry. Before utilizing your shea butter in your intended applications, you can gently rewarm it between your palms or melt it using the double boiler method if it gets too firm.

You may completely utilize the advantages of shea butter in your daily life by investigating these useful applications and ideas. Take advantage of the hydration, nourishment, and adaptability that shea butter offers to your self-care routine.

Chapter 14

The Future of Shea Butter: Innovations and Emerging Trends

In this final chapter, we examine the possibilities of shea butter by emphasizing the fascinating developments and new trends that are influencing it. Shea butter maintains a promising position in the beauty and wellness sector as the demand for natural and sustainable skincare solutions keeps growing. Let's take a look at what this amazing element might become in the future.

1. Expanded Research and Scientific Discoveries: Shea butter has long been prized for its folk remedies and purported health advantages. However, current scientific studies are illuminating its characteristics and possible uses in fresh ways. We may anticipate finding additional proof of shea butter's effectiveness as researchers probe deeper into its chemical structure and consider inventive applications for it in cosmetics, drugs, and other industries.

2. Innovations in formulation: As formulation technology develops, we can expect to see the creation of brand-new, cutting-edge shea butter-based goods. Shea butter is anticipated to be used by beauty businesses in a range of sophisticated and targeted skincare formulations, from serums and face oils to advanced skincare formulations that address particular skin issues. Shea butter may be included in these compositions along with other organic components, antioxidants, or active substances to increase its advantages and meet different skincare requirements.

3. Sustainable Sourcing and Ethical Production: The shea butter sector will continue to place a premium on ethical production methods and sustainable sourcing. Consumers are becoming more aware of how their purchases affect the environment and society. Therefore, we may foresee a growing focus on community empowerment programs, eco-friendly extraction techniques, and fair trade partnerships that support the sustainable production of shea butter while protecting ecosystems and enhancing the standard of living of nearby communities.

4. Diversification into Cosmetics and Personal Care: Shea butter is useful for a variety of cosmetic and personal care applications outside of skincare and haircare due to its adaptability. Shea butter is anticipated to appear in a variety of cosmetic items like foundation, lipstick, and mascara as customer preferences shift toward natural and clean beauty. Its nourishing, protecting, and moisturizing qualities make it a desirable ingredient for boosting the effectiveness and advantages of these products.

5. Global Recognition and Market Expansion: Shea butter is becoming more and more well-known outside of its native African markets. Because of its outstanding qualities and adaptability, it is becoming more widely known and valued. We can anticipate seeing the shea butter market continue to grow as beauty and wellness companies from various regions add it to their product lineups. Additionally, this expansion will encourage joint ventures and partnerships between shea butter suppliers, cosmetic companies, and academic institutions, which will result in more creative and environmentally friendly methods.

Shea butter significantly contributes to the cultural history of the communities from where it is obtained, preserving and empowering them. There will be more initiatives to commemorate and maintain the cultural relevance of this ingredient as shea butter demand increases. Brands can work with regional cooperatives and craftsmen to support the traditional ways of making shea butter, preserving cultural knowledge and strengthening local communities through fair trade and job opportunities.

Shea butter is well-positioned to continue its incredible journey as a cherished natural ingredient in the beauty and wellness sector by embracing these next trends and advances. It is a wonderful gem of nature, providing a plethora of advantages for our skin, hair, and general wellbeing thanks to its lengthy history, sustainable potential, and wide range of applications.

May you continue to benefit from the nourishing and transformational power of this amazing natural ingredient as we explore shea butter's health advantages.

CONCLUSION

Shea butter is a genuine gift from nature that improves our lives in a variety of ways while also providing a wealth of health advantages.
We have examined the extraordinary natural ingredient's rich history, qualities, and wide range of uses in this thorough investigation of shea butter and its health advantages. Shea butter's nourishing, moisturizing, and therapeutic qualities have enthralled people all over the world from its African origins to its current level of appeal.

We started by learning about the shea tree, the traditional techniques of extraction, and processing, as well as the history of shea butter. We looked into the ingredients of shea butter and learned that it has a lot of vital fatty acids, vitamins, and antioxidants, which is why it has so many health benefits.

We looked at the amazing things shea butter can do for our skin, hair, and general health throughout the book. Shea butter has been shown to be a flexible and powerful natural therapy, with benefits ranging from its moisturizing and anti-aging qualities to its capacity to reduce inflammation and speed up wound healing.

The specific advantages of shea butter for various skin and hair disorders, such as dryness, eczema, acne, and frizz, were also covered. It is suitable for all skin types, especially sensitive and delicate skin, due to its gentle and non-comedogenic nature.

Additionally, we looked at the cultural and socioeconomic importance of shea butter, acknowledging its contribution to community empowerment, particularly for women who are frequently active in its production.The significance of using sustainable sourcing and production methods was emphasized in order to protect the environment and guarantee the long-term availability of shea butter.

We investigated new developments and trends in the shea butter sector as we looked to the future. Shea butter is prepared to continue its extraordinary journey as a cherished natural ingredient, thanks to expanded research, scientific advancements, formulation improvements, and market expansion.